Trimming the Fat:

"Strategies, Techniques, and Tips for Achieving Your Ideal Body Composition"

By

Dr James M. Mauldin

Table of contents

Introduction

"Cutting back the Excess" is a convincing and useful manual for accomplishing a solid way of life by rolling out down-to-earth improvements to your dietary patterns. In the present speedy world, it's not difficult to fall into the snare of eating food sources that are high in fat, sugar, and calories, which can prompt weight and an assortment of related medical conditions. In any case, fortunately, it's never past the point where it is possible to begin rolling out certain improvements that can work on your well-being and prosperity.

In this book, you'll find functional tips and methodologies for decreasing your fat admission without forfeiting taste and happiness. From figuring out how to peruse food names and pursuing better food decisions to integrating more activity into your everyday daily practice, "Cutting back the Excess" gives you the information and apparatuses you want to make the enduring way of life changes.

With an abundance of exploration and master guidance, this book is an imperative asset for anybody hoping to work on their well-being and prosperity through better sustenance. Whether you're hoping to shed pounds, lessen your gamble of persistent sickness, or feel improved in your skin, "Cutting

Back the Excess" is a definitive manual for rolling out enduring improvements that will assist you with accomplishing your objectives. So why pause? Begin your excursion to a better you today, and find the groundbreaking force of smart dieting and living!

Chapter 1

Understanding Muscle versus fat

Muscle versus fat is a fundamental part of our body organization, alongside muscle, bone, and organs. It is a put-away type of energy that our body utilizes during times of low food consumption or actual work. While some muscle-to-fat ratio is fundamental for ordinary physical processes, extreme sums can prompt negative well-being outcomes.

The muscle-to-fat ratio can be characterized into two sorts: fundamental fat and stockpiling fat.

Fundamental fat is expected for ordinary physiological capabilities, like managing internal heat levels, padding organs, and delivering chemicals. Capacity fat, then again, is put away in fat tissue and fills in as energy savings for the body.

The sum and circulation of muscle versus fat can differ enormously between people. The muscle-to-fat ratio can be estimated utilizing different strategies, including skinfold thickness estimations, bioelectrical impedance investigation, and double energy X-beam absorptiometry (DXA) filters.

The abundance of muscle versus fat has been connected to various well-being chances, including cardiovascular infection, type 2 diabetes, hypertension,

And a few tumors. The conveyance of muscle versus fat is additionally significant, as people with more instinctive fat (fat put away around the organs) are at a higher gamble of unexpected problems contrasted with those with more subcutaneous fat (fat put away under the skin).

In general, understanding muscle to fat ratio and its job in the body is fundamental for keeping up with great well-being and forestalling negative well-being outcomes related to an abundance of muscle versus fat.

The Rudiments of Muscle to Fat ratio

The muscle-to-fat ratio is a fundamental part of the human body, as it directs internal heat levels, pad organs, and gives a wellspring of energy to the body. In any case, an abundance of muscle versus fat can likewise have negative well-being results.

Muscle versus fat is made out of fat tissue, which is comprised of cells called adipocytes. Adipocytes store energy as fatty substances, which can be separated and utilized for energy when the body needs it.

The muscle versus fat ratio is the extent of fat according to the absolute body weight. The suggested muscle versus fat

Ratio fluctuates relying on elements like age, orientation, and movement level. All things considered, in any case, a solid muscle-to-fat ratio for men is between 10-20%, while for ladies, it is between 20-30%.

It's critical to take note that not everything muscle versus fat is made equivalent. There are two kinds of muscle versus fat: subcutaneous and instinctive. Subcutaneous fat is tracked down underneath the skin and is answerable for the "pinchable" fat in regions like the thighs, hips, and tummy. Instinctive fat, then again, is found somewhere inside the mid-region, encompassing organs like the liver, pancreas, and digestion tracts. This kind of fat is more hazardous to well-being,

As it has been connected to an expanded chance of coronary illness, type 2 diabetes, and other ailments. Understanding muscle versus fat and its dissemination is a significant stage in overseeing and keeping a solid body weight and general well-being.

The Dangers of Abundance Muscle to fat ratio

Abundance muscle to fat ratio can expand the gamble of various medical problems. A portion of the normal dangers related to an overabundance of muscle versus fat is:

Cardiovascular infections: Abundance of muscle versus fat can build the gamble of coronary illness, stroke, and

Hypertension. Fat amassing in the corridors can prompt the development of plaque, which can limit the supply routes and confine the bloodstream.

Diabetes: Corpulence is a significant gamble factor for type 2 diabetes. Overabundance muscle fat ratio can cause insulin opposition, which can prompt high glucose levels and at last diabetes.

Malignant growth: Stoutness has been connected to an expanded gamble of a few kinds of disease, including bosom, colon, and kidney malignant growth.

Rest apnea: Weight can cause breathing troubles during rest, prompting rest

Apnea. This condition is portrayed by stops in breathing during rest, which can cause daytime weariness and other medical problems.

Joint issues: The abundance muscle to fat ratio can come down on the joints, prompting conditions like osteoarthritis.

Emotional wellness issues: Corpulence can build the gamble of wretchedness and other psychological well-being issues.

By and large, an overabundance of muscle versus fat can fundamentally affect both physical and emotional wellness, featuring the significance of keeping a solid

Muscle to fat Ratio Conveyance and Wellbeing Dangers

Muscle versus fat dissemination is the example wherein muscle to fat ratio is conveyed all through the body. There are two primary kinds of muscle-to-fat ratio dispersion:

Android or apple-molded: This kind of muscle-to-fat ratio dispersion is portrayed by an abundance of fat around the mid-region and abdomen. This sort of fat dispersion is more normal in men and is related to a higher gamble of medical conditions like coronary illness, stroke, and type 2 diabetes.

Gynoid or pear-molded: This sort of muscle-to-fat ratio dissemination is described by an overabundance of fat around the hips, thighs, and rear end. This kind of fat dissemination is more normal in ladies and is by and large viewed as less destructive to wellbeing than android fat appropriation.

Overabundance muscle to fat ratio overall is related to various well-being chances, including:

Coronary illness: Overabundance of muscle-to-fat ratio can expand the gamble of coronary illness by raising pulse and cholesterol levels, and expanding the gamble of creating

Conditions like atherosclerosis (limiting the supply routes).

Type 2 diabetes: The abundance muscle to fat ratio can cause insulin obstruction, which can prompt the advancement of type 2 diabetes.

Rest apnea: Overabundance of muscle-to-fat ratio can prompt the improvement of rest apnea, a condition in which breathing is upset during rest.

Joint issues: The abundance muscle to fat ratio can come down on the joints, which can prompt the improvement of joint issues like joint inflammation.

Certain malignant growths: Abundance muscle versus fat has been connected to an expanded gamble of specific sorts of diseases, including bosom malignant growth, colon disease, and endometrial malignant growth.

It's essential to take note that muscle versus fat dispersion and well-being dangers can shift contingent upon various elements, including age, sex, hereditary qualities, and way of life factors like eating regimen and exercise.

Chapter 2

Nourishment and Weight Reduction

Nourishment assumes a critical part in weight reduction. To get thinner, you want to make a calorie deficiency by consuming fewer calories than you consume. Nonetheless, it's vital to guarantee that you're getting every one of the fundamental supplements your body needs to appropriately work.

One method for making a calorie deficiency is to follow your macronutrient consumption. Macronutrients are the three significant supplements that give calories: carbs,

Proteins, and fats. Each macronutrient has an alternate caloric worth, with carbs and proteins containing 4 calories for every gram and fat containing 9 calories for each gram. By following your macronutrient consumption, you can guarantee that you're consuming the suitable measure of every supplement while as yet keeping a calorie deficiency.

One more significant part of sustenance for weight reduction is dinner arranging. Arranging your feasts ahead of time can assist you with settling on better food decisions and staying away from indiscreet choices that can prompt gorging. Some compelling feast-arranging systems incorporate

Dinner preparation, making a basic food item rundown, and cooking at home.

As well as following macronutrients and dinner arrangements, it's essential to be aware of piece estimates and stay away from exceptionally handled food varieties that are high in calories but low in supplements. All things being equal centers around entire, supplement-thick food sources like natural products, vegetables, lean proteins, and entire grains.

In general, sustenance is a vital part of weight reduction. By making a calorie deficiency through careful eating and following macronutrients, dinner arranging, and settling on good food decisions, you can accomplish your weight reduction objectives while as yet

Giving your body the supplements it necessities to appropriately work. Sustenance assumes an essential part in weight reduction. Devouring the right sorts and measures of food can help people accomplish and keep a sound weight. Here are a few key motivations behind why nourishment is significant for weight reduction:

Calorie Control: To get thinner, people should consume fewer calories than they consume. By settling on quality food decisions and rehearsing segment control, people can make a calorie deficiency, which is fundamental for weight reduction.

Macronutrient Equilibrium: Consuming the right equilibrium of macronutrients - protein, starches, and fat - can help people feel full and fulfilled, which can prompt fewer desires and less indulging. A decent eating routine can likewise assist with saving bulk during weight reduction.

Supplement Thickness: Picking supplement-thick food sources - those that are high in nutrients, minerals, and other useful supplements - can assist people with keeping up with their well-being while at the same time shedding pounds. These food sources can assist with supporting the resistant framework, further develop energy levels, and advance general health.

Practical Propensities: By taking on smart dieting propensities and making a supportable way of life changes, people can keep a sound load over the long haul. A sound eating routine can likewise assist with forestalling ongoing infections, like coronary illness, diabetes, and malignant growth, which are frequently connected to an overabundance of weight.

Generally, nourishment is a critical part of any fruitful weight reduction plan. By pursuing good food decisions, people can accomplish their weight reduction objectives and work on their general well-being and prosperity.

Grasping Macronutrients and Calories

Macronutrients are the three fundamental parts of our eating routine that give energy and are expected by the body in enormous sums. These macronutrients are sugars, proteins, and fat.

Starches give energy and are found in food sources like organic products, vegetables, grains, and sugars. Protein is fundamental for building and fixing tissues and can be found in food varieties like meat, fish, eggs, and vegetables. Fat gives energy and retains specific nutrients, and is found in food sources like oils, nuts, and dairy items.

Calories are a unit of estimation for energy. The quantity of calories in a food or drink demonstrates how much energy it can give to the body. Consuming a greater number of calories than the body needs can prompt weight gain while consuming fewer calories than the body needs can prompt weight reduction.

To get fitter, it is vital to make a calorie shortage by consuming fewer calories than the body consumes everyday exercises and exercise. This shortage can be accomplished by diminishing calorie admission through segment control or picking lower-calorie food sources, and expanding calorie use through work out.

It is likewise vital to keep a reasonable admission of macronutrients for generally speaking well-being and prosperity. The suggested day-to-day admission of macronutrient changes relies upon elements like age, sex, weight, and movement level. Counseling medical services proficient or enlisted dietitians can help decide a proper macronutrient and calorie consumption for individual necessities and objectives.

Successful Dinner Arranging Systems

Successful dinner arranging systems can have a tremendous effect on your

Weight reduction venture. Here are a few helpful hints:

Plan your feasts ahead of time: Take a period consistently to design your dinners for the impending week. This will assist you with remaining focused and try not to pursue hasty choices with regard to food decisions.

Make a reasonable dinner plan: Your feast plan ought to incorporate various quality food varieties from all the significant nutritional categories, including organic products, vegetables, entire grains, lean protein, and sound fats.

Segment control: Remember segment sizes while arranging your dinners. Utilizing more modest plates and allotting servings can assist you with controlling your calorie consumption.

Cook at home: Preparing your dinners at home can assist you with controlling what goes into your food and setting aside your cash.

Clump cooking: Consider group preparing feasts ahead of time to save time during the week. You can prepare bigger amounts of food and part them out for numerous dinners.

Utilize solid cooking strategies: Utilize sound cooking techniques like baking,

Searing, barbecuing, or broiling as opposed to searing.

Pack your own dinners: Set up your feasts ahead of time and pack them to take with you to work or school. This can assist you with staying away from the enticement of cheap food or unfortunate tidbits.

Keep solid tidbits available: Keep sound bites like organic products, vegetables, nuts, and seeds close by to check hunger between dinners.

Remember about hydration: Make a point to drink a lot of water over the course of the day to remain hydrated and assist with processing.

By integrating these dinners arranging systems into your daily practice, you can make good dieting more reasonable and manageable as long as possible.

Chapter 3

Exercise and Weight Reduction

Practice is a significant piece of any get-healthy plan. While sustenance is key for making a calorie shortage, exercise can assist with expanding the calorie shortfall, work on generally speaking wellbeing, and assist with keeping up with weight reduction over the long haul.

Here are a few central issues to remember with regard to exercise and weight reduction:

The Advantages of Activity for Weight Reduction: Exercise can assist with

Expanding the number of calories consumed, which can assist with making a bigger calorie deficiency. Moreover, exercise can assist with further developing bulk and strength, which can assist with expanding digestion and advancing weight reduction after some time.

Making an Activity Plan: With regards to making an activity plan for weight reduction, it's critical to consider factors, for example, wellness level, objectives, and individual inclinations. A blend of cardio and strength preparation is regularly suggested for ideal weight reduction results.

Cardio versus Strength Preparing: While both cardio and strength

Preparing can be helpful for weight reduction, they distinctively affect the body. Cardio helps increment calorie consumption and work on cardiovascular well-being, while strength preparation assists increment with muscling mass and work on metabolic rate.

Integrating Actual work Into Day to day existence: notwithstanding organized workouts, it means quite a bit to track down ways of integrating active work into day-to-day existence. This can incorporate things like using the stairwell rather than the lift, taking a stroll during lunch, or doing family errands.

In general, exercise can be an amazing asset for weight reduction and ought to

Be integrated into any health improvement plan. By making an activity plan that is economical and agreeable, people can work on their well-being and accomplish their weight reduction objectives.

Making an Activity Plan

Making an activity plan is a significant stage in any weight reduction venture. Here are a few key contemplations while fostering your arrangement:

Begin with your objectives: What is it that you need to accomplish through a workout? Is it true that you are hoping to develop fortitude, work on cardiovascular well-being, or basically

Consume calories? Realizing your objectives will assist you with fitting your arrangement to meet your particular requirements.

Consider your wellness level: In the event that you're new to working out, it's essential to begin gradually and progressively develop your wellness level. Assuming that you're more capable, you might have to move with additional serious exercises to keep gaining ground.

Pick exercises you appreciate: Exercise doesn't need to be a task. Pick exercises that you appreciate, whether it's running, cycling, moving, or playing

Sports. This will make it almost certain that you stay with your arrangement.

Stir it up: Assortment is critical to forestall fatigue and to challenge your body in various ways. Attempt various kinds of activities, for example, strength preparation, cardio, and adaptability work.

Plan your exercises: Treat your activity plan like some other arrangement and timetable it into your day. This will assist you with remaining responsible and guarantee that you set aside a few minutes for work out.

Consider a fitness coach or wellness class: In the event that you're new to exercise or need some additional inspiration, consider working with a

Fitness coach or taking a wellness class. These can give direction and backing to assist you with arriving at your objectives.

Keep in mind, the way to progress with an activity plan is consistency. Find exercises you appreciate and make them a normal piece of your daily schedule, and you'll be headed to a better, fitter you.

The Advantages of Activity for Weight Reduction

A normal activity offers various advantages for weight reduction, including:

Expanded calorie consumption: Exercise consumes calories and makes a

Calorie deficiency, which is fundamental for weight reduction.

Worked on metabolic rate: Exercise can expand your metabolic rate, which is the rate at which your body consumes calories. This implies that even after your exercise is finished, your body will keep on consuming calories at a higher rate.

Diminished muscle-to-fat ratio: Standard activity can assist you with losing muscle-to-fat ratio, particularly when joined with a sound eating regimen.

Saved bulk: When you get fitter, you ordinarily lose both fat and muscle.

Notwithstanding, ordinary activity can assist with protecting bulk, which is significant for keeping a sound digestion.

Diminished hazard of ongoing infection: Exercise has been displayed to lessen the gamble of persistent sicknesses, like sort 2 diabetes, coronary illness, and particular kinds of disease.

Further developed temperament: Exercise can assist with working on your mindset and diminish pressure, which can be helpful for general well-being and weight the board.
Generally, practice is a significant part of a solid way of life and can be

Extraordinarily gainful for weight reduction. In any case, it's memorable's essential that practice alone isn't enough for weight reduction and should be joined with a sound eating routine and another way of life changes.

Cardio versus Strength Preparing

Cardio and strength preparation are two well-known sorts of activity that offer unmistakable advantages for generally speaking well-being and wellness. Here is a short outline of each:

Cardio:
Cardio, short for cardiovascular activity, is any kind of activity that gets your pulse up and expands your

breathing rate. Models incorporate running, cycling, swimming, and moving. Cardio is incredible for working on cardiovascular well-being, consuming calories, and expanding perseverance. It can likewise further develop a state of mind and diminish feelings of anxiety.

Strength Preparing:
Strength preparing, otherwise called opposition preparing, includes utilizing loads or other protection from fabricated muscle. Models incorporate weightlifting, bodyweight activities, and obstruction band preparation. Strength preparation is astounding for expanding bulk and strength, working on bone thickness, and helping digestion. It can

likewise assist with further developing equilibrium and forestalling wounds.

With regard to weight reduction, both cardio and strength preparation can be successful. Cardio assists with consuming calories, while strength preparation can increment bulk and digestion, prompting more calories consumed very still. A blend of the two kinds of activity is for the most part suggested for ideal well-being and wellness.

Chapter 4

Way of life Changes for Weight reduction

Way of life changes assumes an urgent part in weight reduction and weight the executives. Here is some viable way of life changes that can assist you with getting more fit:

Focus on rest: Getting sufficient rest (7-8 hours in the evening) can assist with controlling chemicals connected with appetite and digestion.

Oversee pressure: Constant pressure can increment cortisol levels, which can

Prompt weight gain. Track down ways of overseeing pressure, like reflection, yoga, or profound breathing activities.

Construct solid propensities: Making little, feasible changes to your everyday schedule can assist you with keeping a sound way of life. For instance, using the stairwell rather than the lift, strolling during your mid-day break, or drinking water rather than pop.

Keep away from handled food varieties: Handled food sources are much of the time high in calories, sugar, and unfortunate fats. Center around eating entire, supplement thick food sources like natural products, vegetables, lean protein, and solid fats.

Practice careful eating: Focusing on your appetite signals, eating gradually, and relishing your food can assist you with trying not to indulge and pursue better decisions.

Remain dynamic over the course of the day: Integrate actual work into your everyday daily schedule, like going for a stroll after supper, doing family tasks, or remaining while at the same time working.

Keep in mind, the way of life changes take time and exertion, however, they can prompt enduring weight reduction and a better life.

Rest and Weight Reduction

sleep is a fundamental part of a sound way of life, and it can assume a significant part in accomplishing and keeping a solid weight. At the point when we don't get sufficient rest, our bodies produce a greater amount of the chemical ghrelin, which invigorates hunger, and less of the chemical leptin, which stifles craving. Therefore, we might feel hungrier than expected, particularly for unhealthy, high-fat food varieties. This can prompt indulging and weight gain over the long haul.

Then again, getting sufficient rest can assist with supporting weight reduction endeavors. Satisfactory rest assists with managing yearning and craving

Chemicals, which can make it simpler to adhere to a smart dieting plan. Furthermore, when we are very much refreshed, we have more energy to exercise and pursue solid decisions over the course of the day.

Here are a few ways to further develop your rest propensities and support weight reduction:

Adhere to a reliable rest plan. Head to sleep and awaken simultaneously every day, even at the end of the week.

Make a loosening up sleep time schedule. Foster a normal that assists you with slowing down before bed, like washing up, perusing a book, or paying attention to quieting music.

Keep away from screens before sleep time. The blue light radiated by telephones, tablets, and PCs can disturb rest, so staying away from them for essentially an hour prior to bed is ideal. Establish a climate that welcomes rest. Ensure your room is cool, dull, and calm, and put resources into agreeable bedding and cushions.

Limit caffeine and liquor. These substances can obstruct the best quality, so it's ideal to stay away from them or consume them with some restraint.
By focusing on rest and making solid rest propensities, you can uphold your weight reduction endeavors and work on your general well-being and prosperity.

Stress and Weight Reduction

Stress can essentially affect weight reduction endeavors. At the point when we experience pressure, our bodies discharge the chemical cortisol, which can prompt expanded hunger and desires for fatty food sources. Furthermore, constant pressure can add to aggravation in the body, which can make it more challenging to shed pounds.

Here are far to oversee pressure and backing weight reduction:

Work out: Exercise is a characteristic pressure reliever and can assist with helping mindset and energy levels. Hold

Back nothing 30 minutes of active work most days of the week.

Care procedures: Rehearsing care methods like contemplation, profound breathing, or yoga can assist with decreasing pressure and work on close-to-home prosperity.

Satisfactory rest: Getting sufficient rest is essential for overseeing pressure and supporting weight reduction. Hold back nothing long stretches of rest each evening.

Adjusted diet: Eating a decent eating routine with a lot of natural products, vegetables, entire grains, lean protein, and sound fats can assist with

Overseeing pressure and backing weight reduction.

Taking care of oneself: Getting some margin for taking care of oneself exercises like perusing, cleaning up, or investing energy outside can assist with lessening feelings of anxiety and work on generally speaking prosperity.
By overseeing feelings of anxiety, people can uphold their weight reduction endeavors and work on their general well-being and prosperity.

Propensities and Weight Reduction
Positively! Here are a few propensities that can add to weight reduction:

Careful Eating: Focusing on what you eat and the amount you eat can assist you with controlling your piece measures and abstaining from indulging.

Drinking Sufficient Water: Drinking water can assist with keeping you full and lessen your calorie consumption.

Ordinary Activity: Customary activity helps consume calories, increment digestion, and keep up with bulk.

Arranging Feasts and Bites: Arranging your dinners and tidbits ahead of time can assist you with pursuing better decisions and staying away from drive-eating.

Getting Sufficient Rest: Getting sufficient rest is significant for directing chemicals that control appetite and totality, and can assist with decreasing feelings of anxiety.

Lessening Pressure: Stress can prompt profound eating and undesirable propensities, so tracking down ways of diminishing pressure can assist you with keeping a sound weight.

Following Advancement: Keeping tabs on your development, whether it's through a food journal or a wellness application, can assist you with remaining responsible and persuasive.

Encircling Yourself with Help: Encircling yourself with strong loved ones who energize sound propensities can assist you with remaining focused and accomplishing your weight reduction objectives.

Chapter 5

Remaining Roused and Staying Away from Mishaps

Here are a few methods for remaining roused and staying away from mishaps while attempting to accomplish weight reduction objectives:

Put forth Reasonable Objectives: Set practical, reachable objectives that line up with your way of life and timetable. Unreasonable objectives can prompt dissatisfaction and disillusionment, which can impede your inspiration.

Observe Little Wins: Praise each little achievement, for example, losing a pound or squeezing into a more modest size. This will assist you with remaining propelled and positive in the meantime.

Find a Responsibility Accomplice: Collaborate with a companion, relative, or mentor to assist with keeping you responsible and spurred. Having somebody to impart your advancement to can assist you with keeping focused.

Keep tabs on Your Development: Track your advancements, like your weight, estimations, and food admission. Seeing the improvement you have made can rouse you to continue onward.

Reward Yourself: Prize yourself with non-food treats for arriving at achievements. This could be another outfit or a spa day.

Stir Up Your Daily Practice: Assortment is vital to keeping away from weariness and remaining spurred. Stir up your workout daily practice and attempt new sound recipes.

Get ready for Misfortunes: Mishaps are ordinary, yet it's critical to have an arrangement set up to defeat them. Recognize your triggers and foster an arrangement to manage them.

Remain Positive: Keep an inspirational perspective and don't allow difficulties

To beat you down. Recall that progress makes time and each little stride combines with your objective.

Defining Sensible Objectives

Putting forth reasonable objectives is a significant piece of any weight reduction venture. At the point when you put forth reasonable objectives, you are bound to stay with your arrangement and accomplish your ideal outcomes. Here are a few ways to define reasonable objectives:

Begin with little objectives: As opposed to laying out a huge objective that might appear to be overpowering, begin with more modest objectives that are simpler

To accomplish. For instance, rather than defining an objective to shed 50 pounds, put forth an objective to shed 5 pounds in the following month.

Be explicit: Ensure your objectives are explicit and quantifiable. Rather than saying you need to "get fitter," put forth an objective to "shed 10 pounds in the following 2 months."

Set a course of events: Give yourself a particular timetable to accomplish your objective. This will assist with keeping you engaged and roused. For instance, put forth an objective to shed 10 pounds in the following 2 months.

Make your objectives sensible: Be straightforward with yourself about what you can reasonably accomplish. In the event that you put forth an objective that is excessively troublesome or unreasonable, you might become deterred and surrender.

Comment on your victories: When you accomplish an objective, find an opportunity to praise your prosperity. This will assist with keeping you roused and zeroed in on your next objective.
Keep in mind, putting forth practical objectives is a significant piece of any weight reduction venture. By setting little, explicit, and attainable objectives, you can gather speed and accomplish your ideal outcomes over the long run.

Conquering Levels and Slowing down

Here are a few potential subjects that could be shrouded in a part on conquering levels and slow down in weight reduction:

Grasping levels and slows down: what they are, the reason they occur, and how lengthy they ordinarily last

Normal reasons for levels and slows down: include physiological variables (for example changes in digestion), mental elements (for example loss of inspiration), and ecological elements (for example changes in the daily schedule or admittance to food)

Systems for getting through levels and slows down: including both dietary and exercise draw near. Models could include:

Calorie cycling or "refeeding" to support digestion and forestall transformation to a low-calorie diet

Consolidating all the more stop-and-go aerobic exercise (HIIT) or different types of "muscle disarray" to challenge the body in new ways

Changing macronutrient proportions or feast timing to all the more likely help weight reduction

Adapting to dissatisfaction and frustration: recognizing that weight reduction isn't generally a direct interaction, and giving methodologies to keeping up with inspiration and point of view during troublesome periods

Knowing when to look for proficient assistance: when levels or slows down persevere in spite of your earnest attempts, it could be an ideal opportunity to talk with a medical care supplier or enrolled dietitian to recognize fundamental causes and foster a more designated strategy.

Dealing with Mistakes and Keeping Up with Progress

Here are a few ways to deal with mistakes and keep up with progress:

Try not to pound yourself: It's memorable's vital that mistakes are an ordinary piece of the weight reduction

Venture. Be caring to yourself and don't allow difficulty to wreck your advancement.

Ponder what occurred: Find an opportunity to consider what caused the goof. Was it an upsetting day at work? Did you surrender to a hankering? Understanding the underlying driver can assist you with staying away from comparative circumstances later on.

Refocus: Don't give one oversight go access to an out-and-out gorge. Refocus on your sound propensities as quickly as time permits.

Put forth little objectives: Setting little, reachable objectives can assist you with

Remaining spurred and centered. Praise your advancement, regardless of how little.

Track down help: Having an emotionally supportive network can have a significant effect with regard to weight reduction. Contact companions, family, or a care group for support and responsibility.

Practice taking care of oneself: Deal with yourself both actually and inwardly. Get sufficient rest, practice pressure-diminishing procedures, and set aside a few minutes for exercises that give you pleasure.

Try not to surrender: Recall that weight reduction is an excursion, not an objective. Try not to abandon yourself, in any event, whenever troubles arise. Continue to push forward and praise each triumph en route.

Conclusion

Congrats! By perusing this book, you have ventured out towards accomplishing a better, more joyful life. You have taken in the fundamentals of muscle-to-fat ratio, the dangers of abundance muscle versus fat, and the significance of sustenance, exercise, and way of life changes for weight reduction.

Be that as it may, shedding pounds is just the initial step. Keeping a sound way of life for life requires continuous responsibility and devotion. Here are a few hints to assist you with keeping focused:

Remain Predictable: Consistency is key with regard to keeping a sound way of life. Adhere to your smart dieting and exercise propensities in any event, when you don't feel like it.

Put forth Practical Objectives: Laying out reasonable objectives for yourself is significant. Try not to attempt to lose an excessive amount of weight excessively fast, or you might become deterred and surrender.

Monitor Your Advancement: Keep a diary or utilize the following application to screen your advancement. This can assist you with remaining spurred and distinguishing regions where you want to get to the next level.

Encircle Yourself with Help: Encircle yourself with steady loved ones who will support and rouse you.

Remain Dynamic: Exercise doesn't need to be a task. Find exercises you appreciate, whether it's moving, climbing, or playing a game, and integrate them into your everyday practice.

Indulge Yourself: Permit yourself to enjoy balance. It's vital to appreciate life and not feel denied.

Keep in mind, a sound way of life is certainly not a transient fix, it's a drawn-out obligation to your well-being and prosperity. With the information and apparatuses you've acquired from this book, you have the ability to roll

Out certain improvements in your day-to-day existence and keep up with them into the indefinite future. Best of luck on your excursion toward a better, more joyful you!